The Practi

Francele Nogueira Moreira
Ingrid Marques
Iara Raquel Castro

The Practice of Nursing Care in Stomatherapy

An approach to stomatherapy and the roles of the stomatherapist

ScienciaScripts

This book is a translation from the original published under ISBN 978-613-9-62381-5.

Publisher:
Sciencia Scripts
is a trademark of
Dodo Books Indian Ocean Ltd. and OmniScriptum S.R.L publishing group

120 High Road, East Finchley, London, N2 9ED, United Kingdom
Str. Armeneasca 28/1, office 1, Chisinau MD-2012, Republic of Moldova, Europe

ISBN: 978-620-7-27636-3

1

I dedicate this work to God, family and friends.

ACKNOWLEDGMENTS

To God who allowed all this to happen, without whom none of this would have been possible and not just in these years as a university student, but at every moment of my life He is my refuge and strength, a very present help in trouble (Psalms 46:1).

To my beloved parents, Maria da Soledade and Claudiomir, for their love, encouragement and for believing and investing in me, supporting me at all times.

To my dear brothers, Michele, Claudiomir and Claudemir, for their brotherhood and unconditional support whenever I needed it.

To my boyfriend, Luis Jeronimo, who in a special and loving way gave me strength and courage, supporting me in times of difficulty and showing me optimism and confidence.

To all the teachers who accompanied me during my undergraduate studies and who contributed greatly to my academic development. To Shirley, the stomatherapist nurse, for her willingness to contribute to the preparation of this work.

To my friends and colleagues for their constant encouragement and support. In particular, my dear friends Dorileudes, Ingrid, Iara Raquel, Genitelma and Rafaella, my work companions who helped me and contributed to my education, are people I keep in my heart and who will always be with me.

To my fellow students Ingrid and Lara Raquel, who joined forces with me to complete this work, for all their hard work and dedication.

I would like to thank everyone who has contributed directly or indirectly to my education.

FRANCELE DA COSTA NOGUEIRA

To God for giving me the gift of life, the strength to overcome difficulties and for giving me wisdom in my choices and allowing all this to happen throughout my life.

To my parents for their encouragement and unconditional love. I would especially like to thank my mother Lucinete, the reason for my life, for giving me support and encouragement in difficult times of discouragement and tiredness, but who, despite the difficulties, never made any effort to help me achieve my dream of becoming a nurse.

I would like to thank my grandmother Juliana for her love and encouragement and for her trust and commitment to my dream, thank you for your companionship and friendship.

To my father Galdino, who, despite his efforts and difficulties, encouraged me and wanted to see me graduate, but unfortunately he is no longer with us.

I would like to thank my brothers and nephews who, in the moments of my life dedicated to my studies, have always made me understand that the future is made up of our choices and efforts dedicated to the present, and have encouraged me in difficult times when I thought I wouldn't make it.

I would like to thank my boyfriend Santiago for being with me from the beginning of this journey, for giving me strength and encouragement when I needed it, and for his companionship and dedication, for always being by my side, always willing to help me.

To my friends Liane Sousa, Werbeth Serejo, and especially to my work companions Francele Nogueira, Ingrid Marques, Rafaella de Castro, Dorileudes Carvalho, Janne Pires, sisters in friendship who were part of my formation and who will certainly continue to be present in my life.

IARA RAQUEL CANTANHEDE CASTRO

First of all to God for giving me the gift of life, health, wisdom, the courage to fight and the perseverance to win.

To my grandparents, parents, aunts and uncles, friends, siblings and cousins, all of whom are part of this achievement. To my group friends: Francele, Iara, Genitelma (Janne), Dorileudes (Dorinha) and Rafaella, who have always been there for me, who have shared every moment since the beginning of my journey and for life.

To the teachers for providing me with knowledge and inspiration during my professional training.

To my study companions: Francele and Iara for their friendship and for being part of this journey and who will remain present in my life.

And to all those who, directly or indirectly, have been part of this journey with encouragement, advice, strength and for believing in me, my thanks.

INGRID MARQUES MENDES

SUMMARY

Stomatherapy is a nursing specialty that promotes preventive and rehabilitative care for people with stomas, acute and chronic wounds, anal and urinary incontinence and fistula. With this in mind, the question arose as to what the practices of stomatherapy care would be for the nursing professional, and the technical skills of the stomatherapy nurse (ET), their main functions and their autonomy in the position were addressed. The aim of this study was to describe the practice of nursing care in enterostomal therapy through a literature review. The scarcity of research on stomatherapy prompted an exploratory study to analyze scientific production on this topic. The study was a descriptive bibliographic review with a qualitative approach that sought to analyze the care practices of ET nurses. The research was based on virtual data from literature search sites such as Google Scholar, Latin American and Caribbean Literature in Health Sciences (LILACS), the Scientific Electronic Library Online (SciELO), the SOBEST website, ESTIMA magazine and books. Among the articles analyzed were those from 2003 to 2017, in Portuguese, available on Integra for online access using the descriptors: stomatherapy, history of stomatherapy, stomatherapy care, nursing. The results of the research show that nurses are technically competent health care professionals with specific skills to perform their duties as enterostomal therapists. In this way, this study aims to provide health professionals with reflections on the field of action, the origin and evolution, as well as the main care of the ET nurse, demonstrating its importance in the process of preventing the loss of skin integrity as well as contemplating holistic care for the human being in its fullness.

Keywords:　　Stomatherapy; History of stomatherapy; Stomatherapy care stomatherapy; Nursing.

SUMMARY

1 INTRODUCTION

Over time, concern about the physical integrity of the skin and the treatment of wounds has become an important part of human health care. There was a search for more knowledge and practices to help restore skin health, which made it even more necessary for a specialized professional to treat wounds, thus giving rise to stomatherapy in nursing (FERREIRA, CANDIDO, CANDIDO, 2010).

Today there is a wide variety of dressings and coverings on the market for the treatment of chronic and complex wounds, as well as a wide variety of devices to help ostomized patients and patients with incontinence, all of which requires a qualified professional who knows how to use all these materials correctly.

In the history of nursing, the profession has gained space and autonomy in wound care, becoming more technical and specific, taking on new responsibilities and competencies in the patient care process. They need to assess and indicate the appropriate dressings, make important decisions regarding treatment and offer support and emotional support to the patient (FERREIRA, CANDIDO, CANDIDO, 2010).

Stomatherapy is a specialty of nursing that covers preventive and rehabilitative care for people with stomas, acute and chronic wounds and anal and urinary incontinence. It is an area of nursing that aims to improve the patient's quality of life by offering holistic and therapeutic care. The stomatherapist nurse (ET) is the trained professional who will provide care to maintain the integrity of the skin (COSTA; BRITO; COSTA, 2013).

It is the specialist who has the autonomy to promote systematized consultations, evaluate and analyze on an ongoing basis, give guidance on dietary care, has the technique to perform specific dressings and, if necessary, refer to other professionals, contributing to multi-professional care and guaranteeing the quality of care. It is of the utmost importance that professionals are retrained to update their knowledge and techniques (YAMADA et al, 2009).

The historical development of stomatherapy began in 1961, when the first stomatherapists were trained around the world. In Brazil, specialization only took place in 1990, with Vera Lucia C.G. Santos standing out as the forerunner of the course in Brazil. In 1992, the Brazilian Society of Stomatherapy (SOBEST) was created, helping to regulate the course and further spread specialization in the country (DIAS, PAULA, MORITA, 2014).

SOBEST will base the ethical and legal aspects of the professional practice of stomatherapy with the aim of bringing together all professionals, training them with standardized teaching, promoting continuous improvement, to ensure the quality of education in stomatherapy. An important milestone was the creation of ESTIMA magazine, an important tool for updating professionals (DIAS, PAULA, MORITA, 2014).

Studies show that there is a positive influence of ET care on the recovery of patients in various parts of the world (BORGES, 2016). This raises the question of what stomatherapy practices would be for nursing professionals and, in view of this problem, the answer will be to address the technical skills of ET nurses, their main functions and their autonomy in the position.

It is a nursing specialization that is on the rise. The trajectory of stomatherapy in the country has come a long way and today it is much more widespread and there are several places that offer the course to specialize. It is now recognized that wound care and the proper use of dressings, as well as the choice of dressing, is the responsibility of the ET.

It is essential to understand that patients with wounds, ostomies and incontinence need differentiated care, requiring professionals to have a broader knowledge of stomatherapy care practices. For this reason, it is essential to carry out studies and research on the subject in order to develop and expand devices to ensure the best care for users.

The relevance of this work lies in the possibility of contributing to improving the quality of care provided to patients with wounds, stomas or incontinence by health professionals, especially ET professionals, with a view to providing more qualified care. It also highlights the autonomy of the professional, as well as clarifying their main skills in the rehabilitation process of the stoma patient.

This research is justified in order to contribute to the knowledge of health professionals, especially nurses, on the proposed topic, since nurses are the professionals who deal directly with wound care. Within this context, this study summarizes the main nursing care of ET. It also emphasizes the nurse's conduct to ensure excellent care.

The scarcity of research on stomatherapy prompted an exploratory study to analyze scientific production on this topic. This is a descriptive bibliographic review study with a qualitative approach that analyzes nursing care practices in stomatherapy.

This research selected articles based on virtual data from literature search sites and books. We used studies found on Google Scholar, Latin American and Caribbean Literature in Health Sciences (LILACS), the Scientific Electronic Library Online (SciELO), the SOBEST website, Revista Estima over the last fourteen years (2003 - 2017).

Data collection was carried out by students from July 2016 to April 2017. 41 articles and 3 books were found. The following words were used as descriptors: stomatherapy, history of stomatherapy, stomatherapy care, nursing.

Of these articles analyzed, only twenty-six met the criteria established based on titles and abstracts for obtaining results and discussion, which were articles published from 2003 to 2017 and which met the objectives of the proposed theme. The articles were organized in a database where they were selected and read in full.

To prepare this literature review, the following steps were taken: definition of the guiding question (problem) and research objectives; establishment of inclusion and exclusion criteria for the publications (sample selection); literature search; analysis and categorization of the studies, presentation and discussion of the results.

This study included articles published from 2003 to 2017, indexed in the selected databases in Portuguese, which addressed the historical milestones of stomatherapy, the main competencies and care of ET nurses. Publications published before 2003 that did not meet the proposed objectives were not included in this study.

In this way, this study aims to provide health professionals with a reflection on the field of action, the origin and evolution, as well as the main care of the ET nurse, demonstrating its importance in the process of preventing the loss of skin integrity.

1.1. Research Problem

What is the practice of nursing care in stomatherapy?

1.2. Objectives

General:

Identify the role of nurses in stomatherapy support in scientific productions.

Specifics:

- Describe the origin and historical evolution of stomatherapy;
- Identify the role of the stomatherapist nurse;
- Describe the nursing care of the stomatherapist.

2 HISTORY AND EVOLUTION OF STOMATHERAPY

The specialty of stomatherapy originated along with the history of medicine, and from then on some terms derived from Greek defined what ostomy was, stoma "which means mouth or opening, to indicate the exteriorization of any hollow viscera through the body or for various causes" (SANTOS, 2015, p.1). In ancient times, around 300 BC, writings report that it was Praxagoras who performed the first operations for abdominal trauma (SANTOS, 2015).

Intestinal stomas are characterized by "the exteriorization of the ileum or colon to the external environment through the abdominal wall" (ROCHA, 2011,   p.51). E It's worth remembering that a colostomy "communicates the colon (large intestine) with the outside", an ileostomy "communicates the small intestine with the outside" (MORAIS, 2009, p. 8-9) and a urostomy is a procedure that aims to change the normal route of urine (MORAIS, 2009, p.10).

In 1710, the stoma was idealized through a necropsy examination carried out by Alex Littre, who discovered that the intestine could be exposed and glued to the wall of the abdomen without any loss to the patient. As such, he was considered the "father of the colostomy" (SANTOS, 2015).

The first colostomy surgery that has been reported in history generates some doubts, as there are reports from 1750 that it was performed on a woman with an incarcerated hernia, but there are also reports that point to Pillore as the first to perform the first ostomy operation (SANTOS, 2015).

As stated by Zampire and Jatoba (apud SANTOS, 2015, p.2):

> The flap colostomy with a support pole was introduced by Maydl in 1883, while the colostomy with two mouths separated by skin segments was proposed by Block in 1892 and by Witzel in 1894. At the turn of the century, the Paul and Miculiez technique proposed the "rifle barrel" colostomy in which the distal and proximal flaps are arranged parallel to each other and perpendicular to the abdominal wall. Thus, the first ileostomy on record was made in 1879, and many years later Baum performed surgery as a form of temporary bypass on a patient with obstructive cancer of the ascending colon who died. The first patient to survive after the ileostomy procedure was reported by Maydl, from Austria, in 1883, also operated on for colon cancer.

In 1930, an ileostomy was exteriorized from the main surgery performed by surgeon McBurney. From then on, new ideas emerged, as in the same period Alfredo A. Strauss made the first collection bag for ileostomized patients, which was later perfected by a chemistry student called Koening (SANTOS, 2015).

"The device was made of adherent rubber that covered the stoma, preventing the contents from leaking through to the skin and fixed to it with a latex preparation, as well as containing a device for attaching a belt to increase safety" (SANTOS, 2015, p.3). The system became known as the Strauss Koening Rutzen bag, which was widely accepted in 1940, even with the limitations it still had (SANTOS, 2015).

The year 1950 saw the development of equipment and surgery in the area of ostomies. In London, Brooke and in Cleveland, Turnbull proposed the total alteration of the ileal mucosa. This technique is still used today and contributes greatly to the overall well-being of the individual (SANTOS, 2015).

As a result, the number of publications on ostomized patients has grown increasingly. Not only referring to surgical techniques, but also including the post-operative period and also providing pertinent information on sexuality, odor control, pregnancy and rehabilitation (SANTOS, 2015).

According to the above, new techniques were employed after Turnbull and Brooke's discovery. To contain all types of ostomy, both intestinal and urinary, Kock bags were created for ileostomies and urostomies, and colostomies were contained with muscular and magnetic rings (SANTOS, 2015).

In 1952, Turnbull accidentally discovered the greatest technological advance ever used at the time, which was Karaya powder. This means "gum with absorbent power", extracted from a tree found in India. After being used on several patients, it showed excellent results (SANTOS, 2015).

Because of the great effectiveness of gum, Turnbull contacted a chemical engineer called Leonard Fenton to produce a bag with a ring of this product so that it could be used in the post-operative phase. From this, "the first peristomal skin barrier was instituted, revolutionizing ostomy care" (SANTOS, 2015, p.4).

It was found that despite the evolution of stoma surgery in terms of care, there were still precarious conditions and the collection systems were also flawed. Thus, those who survived after surgery were isolated from society, did not work, and were unhappy (SANTOS, 2015).

As previously mentioned, due to the lack of knowledge about caring for colostomized patients in terms of their physical, mental and social health, the first publication on the subject of "care for ostomized patients" was by Du Bois, in the American Journal of Nursing, where the author discusses nutrition, self-care, the location of the stoma, among other related factors (SANTOS, 2015).

At the beginning of the evolution of nursing, from the time when care was provided by religious people to the modern era, with the pioneer of nursing Florence Nightingale, many theories were created and since then there has been a time of discovery and new techniques. The profession also grew along with technological advances and sought new paths that required more specific knowledge and skills to improve its practice (DIAS, PAULA, MORITA, 2014).

According to Dias, Paula and Morita (2014), the history of stomatherapy can be separated into two phases: the first phase comprises the ancient age up to 1949 and the second phase comprises the 1950s up to the present day, when it became recognized as a specialty. This first moment began to define the general profile of stomatherapy, which also includes two events: "the evolution of surgical techniques for stomas and the creation of devices for use by people with stomas". The second moment saw the creation of groups of people with stomas, as well as the advancement of technological devices.

In 1955, Danish nurse Elise Sorense created the first pouch for stoma patients, contributing to the first nursing report on stoma care. Even then, it was clear that the stoma patient had many other needs besides surgery; special attention was needed for their rehabilitation, which included post-operative care as well as aspects of sexuality, care for skin integrity and the correct handling of the bag (DIAS, PAULA, MORITA, 2014).

With all these events, surgeon Rupert Turnbull hired Norma Gill, who was ileostomized and had experience in the field, having looked after her colostomized grandmother for two years, to work with him as a stoma technician (YAMADA, ROGENSKI, OLIVEIRA, 2003). Other factors should also be considered besides the location of the bag, such as the physical and emotional well-being of the person with the ostomy.

The specialty of stomatherapy is a recent one, officially born in 1961 at the Cleveland Clinic Foundation - in the United States of America, being instituted as the first course in the world (YAMADA, digital text). It went on to train nurses in the performance of care and students who were stomatized.

Some important milestones were the founding of the first organization of enterostomal therapists through the North American Association of Enterostomal Therapists (NAAET) in 1968, as well as the emergence of the International Association for Enterostomal Therapy (IAET) in 1971, which is currently the Wound, Ostomy and

Continence Nursing Society - WOCN (DIAS, PAULA, MORITA, 2014).

2.1 History of Stomatherapy in Brazil

Although we know that the beginning of stomatherapy in Brazil was made official with the specialization course in nursing, there were other movements in other countries that contributed to its development and expansion. In Canada and the USA, in the 1970s, they created a new way of organizing care for ostomates, in terms of care and more appropriate devices. Professionals from various fields, especially nurses, mobilized to improve their technical and scientific skills (SANTOS, 2015).

As a result, in the 1980s, nursing professionals traveled to countries such as the USA, Colombia and Spain to specialize their training and when they returned they contributed to the qualification of other professionals as well as motivating them to work with ostomates (SANTOS, 2015).

Alongside these events, "the movement of ostomized people's associations was strengthened with the creation of the Brazilian Society of Ostomized People (SOB), which achieved some goals related to the purchase and distribution of devices" (SANTOS, 2015).

In Brazil, with the advances in stomatherapy, there have been several relevant points in the evolution of the specialty, and in 1961 the first congress was held to train technical skills in stomas. Most of the people who sought this qualification were stoma patients themselves, who needed knowledge and skills focused on the problem at hand, acquiring specific techniques and care (CESARETTI, LEITE, 2015).

In the same year, the Department of Abdominal Stomatherapy was created at the Fergusondroste - Ferguson Hospital, which collaborated with the development of the specialty, with studies seeking to improve the quality of life for stoma patients (CESARETTI, LEITE, 2015).

In 1968, the North American Association of Enterostomal Therapists (NAAET) was created and changed in 1971 to the International Association for Enterostomal Therapy (IAET), which established standards that would lead to nursing providing new studies that would promote quality of life and techniques aimed specifically at nursing (CESARETTI, LEITE, 2015).

With the progress of stomatherapy, there was a great demand for the specialty, with 351 professionals specializing in 1973 with the Health Apprenticeship Program, seeking to qualify professionals. With the increase in the number of professionals trained, they began to be required to have the technical knowledge, scientific theory and skills to provide safe care to ostomized users (CESARETTI, LEITE, 2015).

The Ostomized Club was founded in Fortaleza in 1975. In 1978, the need for a responsible body arose, and the Word Council Of Enterostomal Therapists - An Association Of Nurses (WCET) was created, a body that represented the entire world, that provided an exchange of knowledge between professionals, thus improving their skills and seeking a standard among themselves, with the aim of providing quality care to people with ostomies, wounds and anal and urinary incontinence (DIAS, PAULA, MORITA, 2014).

In 1985, the Brazilian Society of Ostomized People (SOB) was founded and played an important role with the government, helping to distribute and buy bags and other benefits for users, making their lives easier. At the same time, there were important milestones for stomatherapy in the country: The training of the first stomatherapists, the creation of the Specialization Course in Stomatherapy in Nursing and the founding of the Brazilian Society of Stomatherapy: Ostomized, Wounds, Incontinence - SOBEST (DIAS, PAULA, MORITA 2014).

The first stomatherapist nurse in Brazil was Gelse Zerbeto, and Vera Lucia Conceigao de Gouveia Santos, who founded the first specialization course in Brazil, at the University of Sao Paulo - USP (YAMADA, digital text).

The Specialization in Stomatherapy Nursing course has some training aspects that follow guidelines where it must have: a minimum theoretical-practical load of 360 hours, the course can take place full-time, part-time or at a distance, the content of the program must be taught by specialists in the field who must follow the following standardization as: "stomatherapy, nursing, administration, dermatology, gastroenterology, home care and palliative care, nutrition, oncology, pharmacy, medicine (coloproctologist), among others" (YAMADA, ROGENSKI, OLIVEIRA, 2003).

In 1984, there was a small study group that was doing research and making discoveries about ostomies, and so SOBEST was created by students who called themselves at the time the Clinical Interest Group in Stomatherapy Nursing - GICEE (SANTOS, 2015).

With the evolution of stomatherapy, there have been several discoveries about ostomies and many studies on the subject. A congress on ostomies was held and the need for a body responsible for stomatherapy as a specialty was realized. This is why

SOBEST was officially created in Brazil in 1993 (SANTOS, 2015). In 2005, the name Society had to be changed to Association, due to the new Brazilian civil code (DIAS, PAULA, MORITA, 2014).

As the history of stomatherapy has progressed, there have been major improvements in the quality of care, as well as in teaching and research in the area, strengthening the functions of the specialist, as well as characterizing the profile of the ET nurse. It is a specialty that is on the rise and that has a wide job market because it has a diverse range of options to work in, ranging from teaching, consulting, administration and others (DIAS, PAULA, MORITA, 2014).

3 THE ROLE OF THE STOMATHERAPIST NURSE

Since the dawn of nursing, there has been a significant evolution in patient care, as seen since the time of Florence Nightingale. This has influenced the technical and scientific development of specific skills and functions to "prevent health, develop control and decision-making, independence, maintain or rebuild identity for the individual dealing with illness" (SANTOS, 2015, p. 6).

> Stomal Therapist Nurse means a nurse with a specialization (post-graduation latu sensu) in the area, whose courses are recognized by the Brazilian Society of Stomatology (SOBEST) and/or the World Council of Enterostomal Therapists (WCET). These nurses provide assistance to people with stomas, fistulas, tubes, catheters and drains, acute and chronic wounds and anal and urinary incontinence, in preventive, therapeutic and rehabilitation aspects in order to improve quality of life (BRASIL, Ordinance No. 620, 2010).

Specialization is considered to be a means of ensuring professional autonomy in theoretical and practical knowledge, seeking to guarantee better quality in the performance of the function, contributing to increased quality and customer satisfaction (SANTOS, 2015). The professional who has autonomy is the one who manages to dominate their work space, expanding their professional knowledge and remaining confident in their abilities (FERREIRA, CANDIDO, CANDIDO, 2010).

TEs need to be aware that their autonomy is not limited only to choosing the most appropriate method for treatment, but that they must have a holistic view of the patient, helping to meet their basic needs, whether physical, mental or social, because individuals with a wound, stoma or incontinence require global care, requiring differential monitoring (FERREIRA, CANDIDO, CANDIDO, 2010).

Ferreira, Bogamil, Tormenta (2008), as quoted by Costa, Brito, Costa (2013, p.1942), choosing a cover, cream or solution for an injury is an example of the practice of autonomy within nursing, here the professional is able to carry out their promotion, prevention and rehabilitation actions much more efficiently. Nurses should only act in this way if they are technically competent and able to carry out their duties responsibly and independently (FERREIRA, CANDIDO, CANDIDO, 2010).

The meaning of being a specialist in nursing is when the professional graduates in generalist nursing and specializes in a specific field, becoming dominant in the subject. "Specialty practice includes clinical, teaching, administrative, research and consulting roles" (SANTOS, 2015, p.7). Thus, postgraduate study in nursing guarantees the progression of care as well as providing a formal, scientific basis with exclusive competence in the area of specialization (SANTOS, 2015).

With the advent of so many technologies that characterize today's modern society, there is a need for specialized nurses who have comprehensive knowledge and are able to take a more detailed view of care than non-specialist nurses (YAMADA; ROGENSKI; OLIVEIRA, 2003). It is therefore essential that those with an interest in the field of stomatherapy seek specialized training through the competent bodies.

Like any specialty studied, stomatherapy has a model that determines the identity of the professional. This was developed in 1980 by Houle and defines that the professional must have an established function, play a role in solving the problems encountered, as well as committing to their own decisions. In this sense, building together with the bodies that represent the profession defines a collective identity (SANTOS, 2015).

TEs therefore need to take ownership of their roles in order to ensure improvements in the individual and collective care they provide, given that their clientele is vast, remembering to always base their actions on scientific knowledge (SANTOS, 2015).

According to Santos (2015, p. 8) the ET has been assigned duties that determine its actions, such as:

> • **care and specialized support function**: encompasses individualized care activities in the immediate, intermediate and late pre- and post-operative phases, aimed at rehabilitation and quality of life based on self-care and integration with the family and the interdisciplinary team as philosophical principles. It involves not only caring for real and potential problems, but also preventative measures and long-term care;
>
> • **educational or teaching function**: includes formal and informal educational activities aimed at the patient, family and community; nurses and nursing and interdisciplinary teams, as well as the development of follow-up protocols and teaching programs, as well as publications;
>
> • **research function**: includes the development of research related to care technology in stomatherapy and the evaluation of care protocols and specific devices (in their improvement and creation);
>
> • **administrative function**: aimed at control and evaluation at the assistance and organizational levels, including the planning and organization of Assistance Programs and Services; planning and distribution of human and material resources, as well as consultancy and advisory services;
>
> • **professional development**: involves participation in continuing education activities, updating and retraining, as well as periodic recertification in specialization.

OT has a vast field of activity that is not limited to caring for the integrity of the skin, for example, but for human beings in all areas of their lives. What's more, the support of a multidisciplinary team is essential, involving not only the patient, but the family as a whole (FERREIRA, CANDIDO, CANDIDO, 2010).

Stomatherapy is not only defined by the physical care and rehabilitation of the patient. However, care will encompass the values and beliefs of the individual, and it is the responsibility of the professional to ensure that all rights and needs are provided in a complete way to the patient (FERREIRA, CANDIDO, CANDIDO, 2010).

The area of stomatherapy is part of the international system of care, seeking to ensure the full satisfaction of these people in terms of the care and resources offered. Thus, those with special needs have the right to specialized comprehensive care guided by ET (CESARETTI, LEITE, 2015).

"The ET has the dual responsibility of providing specialized care to people with specific needs, as well as sharing skills and knowledge with other professionals" (CESARETTI, LEITE, 2015 p.25).

As this field is little explored, there is a clear need for specialists, which is why research should be encouraged, as well as the availability of training programs. This is so that we can learn more about the specialty and improve the knowledge of professionals who are already qualified to guarantee the care provided (CESARETTI, LEITE, 2015).

Santos (2001 apud PAULA; SANTOS, 2003) says that the ET is a professional with the knowledge and training to exercise skills and techniques in the care of people with ostomies, wounds and incontinence. The specialist has a very large field of action within his reality, but the difficulties are also great in exercising his role within an institution, so it is important to understand what the ET's role is and how he can exercise his skills satisfactorily.

It can be clearly seen that ET has a great significance and is making its way, as it is a growing specialization. The objectives need to be well defined so that a new view of the ET nurse can be gained in society and wherever they are inserted, since they are an exclusive, elementary and crucial professional for the exercise of health in the country (PAULA; SANTOS, 2003).

4 MAIN NURSING CARE FOR STOMATHERAPISTS

4.1.   Stoma area

The word "stoma" is of Greek origin and means "mouth or opening". "It is any exteriorization of hollow viscera, such as trachea, stomach, intestine and urinary tract, with the aim of feeding or eliminating liquids and physiological effluents" (CARVALHO, CARDOSO, 2014, p. 487).

Intestinal stomas are a rupture made in the abdomen which, depending on the location, can change nomenclature such as: ascending colostomy   : for liquid stools; transverse colostomy: semi-liquid stools;

descending colostomy: feces are formed; sigmoid colostomy: feces are firm and solid. It is performed through a surgical process and is the exposure of the large intestine on the abdominal wall (RODRIGUES et al, 2008).

After the surgical process, many changes begin to appear in the lifestyle of stoma patients. Some patients do not accept the new way of life, because some aspects such as eating, dressing and other personal habits change and this all happens as a consequence of their emotions, anxiety, daily conflicts, physiological and psychosocial problems, their old habits, their values and beliefs, fear of being rejected, all of which contributes to the patient's isolation and can also develop into depression (SOUZA et al, 2012).

Given all these situations experienced by the patient, it can be seen that they are susceptible to many complications if they are not accompanied from the start of treatment, which begins when surgery is indicated. Therefore, qualified assistance is required from a specialized professional such as an ET who must have specific skills for the problems presented here (VASCONCELLOS, XAVIER, 2015).

The ET is the professional capable of assisting these clients and their health actions during care should encourage the patient's autonomy and selflessness, helping them to live a more noble life (SOUZA et al 2012). The ET has the role of helping the stoma bearer to reintegrate into society by drawing up care plans for adaptation and acceptance, because the patient tends to exclude himself from society, and it is necessary to make him accept his new living condition (SOUZA et al 2012).

After surgery, possible complications can occur at the beginning or some time after the operation. "Early complications are: bleeding, swelling, ischemia, detachment, mucocutaneous and late complications are: dermatitis, stenosis, hernia and prolapse" (VASCONCELLOS, XAVIER, 2015, p.28). It is important for the ET to promote health education with the family, explaining everything that can happen to the patient.

"The ET and the nursing team must assist the client in all surgical phases, from the demarcation of the stoma, to its preparation and in the immediate post-operative period with the visualization of it" (VASCONCELLOS, XAVIER, 2015, p.28).

The ET is responsible for carrying out the nursing consultation with stoma patients in the first phase of the preoperative period, where he/she will need to use methods in the assessments that facilitate the systematization of nursing care in stomatherapy, also using instruments in the physical assessment, since it is the nurse's responsibility to locate the surgery, in this phase the professional needs to take into account all the patient's history such as general health, socio-demographic and physical examination (YAMADA et al, 2009).

It is essential to provide the patient with guidance on the surgical procedure and to clarify any doubts they may have, as well as preparing the equipment that will be used, collectors, and carrying out sensitivity tests on the material that will be used (YAMADA et al, 2009).

In the second phase, which is intra-operative, it is necessary to exchange information between the surgeon and the ET in the operating room about the material for each type of stoma that will be used, thus ensuring that the stoma is made in the marked area, thereby reducing the rates of infection and complications (YAMADA et al, 2009).

In the third phase, which is the post-operative period, which can be immediate or immediate, the ET has to make home visits, assessing the appearance of the stoma, the residues that are being eliminated and checking for signs of possible complications, prescribing essential care if there are any and encouraging self-care, helping the family to help the patient, making them aware that they can lead a normal life, thus helping the patient to have a good rehabilitation (YAMADA et al, 2009).

In the late post-operative period, the professional assesses the condition of the skin and the appearance of complications and, if there are any, determines care and equipment in cases of dermatitis, retraction, prolapses and teaches the patient to self-irrigate in order to have a more adequate, quick and effective rehabilitation (YAMADA et al, 2009).

For good, qualified nursing care in the rehabilitation of patients with ostomies, thus reducing the consequences left after surgery and its consequences, the rehabilitation phase is developed by the ET who has to emphasize self-care, know their limits and abilities, teach the patient to face their fears, fantasies, re-establishing their living conditions, which can be reintegrated with appropriate treatments and guidance, through educational projects aimed at the situation of each patient (SOUZA et al, 2012).

The main precautions are: monitoring the stoma area every time the bag is changed, always paying attention to coloration, noticing if the skin is irritated or bruised to avoid necrosis and ischemia, preventing feces from coming into contact with the skin around the stoma, keeping the area clean and sanitizing it with soap and water (RODRIGUES et al, 2008).

Always take note of the changes in the stoma and the appearance of the stool so that you can see if the intestine is functioning properly and if the diet is adapted. Always use collectors that are larger than the size of the stoma so that they cover it completely, thus avoiding the risk of skin lesions (RODRIGUES et al, 2008).

The ET can advise on the most appropriate type of diet so that the intestine works more effectively and more easily for digestion, should help with the patient's self-esteem and advise on sex life, as this is another problem that many face. It is a delicate moment that requires the professional to provide psychological support with guidance and adjustments so that the client and their partner can develop their sexual activities normally (VASCONCELLOS, XAVIER, 2015).

4.2. Wound Area

The skin is an organ whose main function is to protect the organs from external agents. There are various causative agents that can alter the integrity of the skin, resulting in wounds. These factors that can trigger an injury range from pressure on the skin to trauma or surgery (MITTAG et al, 2017).

"A wound is represented by the interruption of the continuity of a bodily tissue, to a greater or lesser extent, caused by any type of physical, chemical or mechanical trauma or triggered by a clinical condition, which activates the organic defense fronts" (BRITO et al, 2013, p.415).

It is known that all attention is essential when it comes to caring for acute or chronic wounds, as it is a complex procedure that requires dynamism (BRITO et al, 2013). "Wounds can be classified as acute or chronic according to the time taken for tissue repair" (FRANQA, et al, 2015, digital text). Chronic wounds are those that are serious and have a rapid evolution time and for their proper treatment the conditions that predispose to normal healing of the wound must be considered (BRITO et al, 2013).

In contrast, "acute wounds are the result of surgery and trauma, where tissue repair occurs in an appropriate sequence and time, without complications, leading to the restoration of anatomical and functional integrity" (FRANQA, et al, 2015, digital text).

Thus, wounds are classified according to the time they appear in the tissue, and when acute, they start suddenly with local pain, but without prolonged suffering because they are short-lived. However, the clinical manifestations of chronic wounds range from functional incapacity to affecting psychosocial changes in the individual (BRITO et al, 2013).

"Preventing, assessing and treating a wound are almost exclusive responsibilities of nursing. It is essential to know the risk factors, physiology, anatomy and the healing process" (MITTAG, et al, 2017, p.20). Therefore, knowing the types of injury and the technological evolution to prevent and treat a wound are fundamental knowledge that should be required by the professional specialized in stomatherapy (MITTAG, 2017).

"The practice of caring for people with wounds is a specialty within nursing, recognized by the Brazilian Society of Dermatology Nursing - SOBEND and the Brazilian Association of Stomatherapy - SOBEST" (BRITO, et al, 2013, p.415). Caring for wounds requires not only knowledge of the area under study, but also specific skills and a comprehensive attitude towards the person with the wound (BRITO, et al, 2013).

There must be a strategy for care in the ET profession in order to obtain a good response in the treatment of skin lesions and their prevention (MITTAG, 2017). When treating wounds, one must understand the evolution of the healing process, as well as the choice of medication (TIMBY, 2007 apud CARNEIRO, SOUSA, GAMA, 2010).

It is the nurse's job to teach the patient to practice self-care, so that the recovery process takes less time. Therefore, this professional is responsible for maintaining the health of the injured area and it is their duty to guide the patient through every procedure to be followed (CARNEIRO, SOUSA, GAMA, 2010). "Evaluating a wound means describing it, recording its characteristics and its evolutionary phase, so that the clinical documentation provides a useful reference in the treatment of wounds" (OROSCO, MARTINS, 2006, p.40).

In order for tissue repair to be satisfactory or not, various reasons, both local and systemic, influence the assessment of the patient and their wound. As wound healing progresses, some factors are taken into account, such as: wound classification, measurement, characteristics of the skin around the wound, degree of infection, characteristics of the tissue in the wound, as well as age, psychological factors, nutrition, among others (OROSCO, MARTINS, 2006).

4.2.1 Nursing Care for Wounds (Pressure Ulcers, Diabetic Wounds, Vasculogenic Wounds of Venous and Arterial Origin, Neurotrophic Wounds due to Hansen's Disease, among others)

"Competence is applying skills in a context that includes assessment, differential diagnosis, development and application of a care plan and its evolution" (FERREIRA, CANDIDO, CANDIDO, 2010,   p.658), so the competent professional in wound care will only be full with the application of the Systematization of Nursing Care - SAE (FERREIRA, CANDIDO, CANDIDO, 2010).

The responsibility for wound care is attributed to the generalist nurse and the ET, and these are set out below:

Carry out nursing consultations with users with wounds (YAMADA et al, 2009). Assess the injured area and the most appropriate treatment should be carried out (CAMPOS, MORE, ARRUDA, 2008). Care should be taken with the skin to preserve its integrity. "Request biochemical and hematological tests, and perform vesico-intestinal re-education when necessary" (YAMADA et al, 2009, digital text).

Guidance should be given on diet and fluid intake, and if necessary, a nutritionist should be asked for an assessment (YAMADA et al, 2009). "Perform instrumental and conservative debridement, wound culture, topical and adjunctive therapy (LASER, electrostimulation, vacuum therapy and others)" (YAMADA et al, 2009, digital text).

In the follow-up of venous ulcer treatment, for example, the costs of procedures should be evaluated, as well as the use of scales as a method of assessing ulcer healing. The professional collects a brief summary of the patient's history regarding the lower limbs. It is of the utmost importance to carry out a physical examination and anamnesis so that a care plan can be drawn up and, consequently, the results of their actions can be analyzed (SILVA et al, 2009).

"Examine the ankle-brachial index using peripheral vascular Doppler. Perform podiatric precautions (nails, cleaning of mycosis, cutting, correction of deformities, removal of spicules)" (YAMADA et al, 2009, digital text). The feet should be well cared for and if there are corns or calluses, they should be removed. Another important measure is to offer emotional and mental support (YAMADA et al, 2009).

Encourage the practice of exercises to strengthen the leg muscles, as well as alternating rest and elevation of the lower limbs. Perform lymphatic drainage and use compressive measures such as the Unna boot or compressive therapy (YAMADA et al, 2009). In the case of leprosy, record the disease/investigation notification form, and later, in order to identify the degree and location of any nerve damage, examine the feet with equipment that makes it easier to detect the problem (YAMADA et al, 2009).

Determining "care and preventive measures for disability, as well as guiding the use of appropriate footwear and insoles" (YAMADA et al, 2009, digital text). Caregivers who are responsible for helping to care for patients with wounds should be guided and supervised by a specialist. When indicated, the nurse should prescribe coverings, solutions or creams for dressing the wounds (CAMPOS, MORE, ARRUDA, 2008).

"Make home visits and draw up opinions, and order complementary tests when necessary, such as: complete blood count, serum albumin, glycemia and exudate culture with antibiogram" (CAMPOS, MORE, ARRUDA, 2008, p.60).

Train the team by offering the necessary training, so that they can establish an approach that satisfies the basic needs of the client and generates up-to-date professionals, as well as providing ongoing education (TEIXEIRA, MENEZES, OLIVEIRA, 2016).

"Forecasting dressing products sent by the monthly resupply request to the resources sector" (CAMPOS, MORE, ARRUDA, 2008, p.57). Being a member of the team that monitors the dressing materials in demand and their dispensation.

In short, the ability to assess an injured area is a nurse's technical competence. Because of this, care should not only be carried out on the wound, but should ensure that this human being is cared for to the full (FERREIRA, CANDIDO, CANDIDO, 2010).

4.3.   Incontinence Area

Incontinence brings major physical and social changes. It is characterized as the loss of the ability to retain or control faeces or urine. Since it is a very common problem, especially in the elderly, nurses are gaining ground in terms of actively participating in the treatment of incontinent patients (HONORIO, SANTOS, 2010).

Caring for any pathology requires the professional providing the service to have a scientific and practical basis. For ET, it's no different: they need to have an understanding of how urinary/anal leakage works, as well as the mechanism of continence and possible treatments for the problem, ranging from surgery to conservative or even pharmacological treatment. They should indicate the most appropriate treatment for each patient, so that they can provide a quality service, helping the patient and their family to make the best choice of treatment (HONORIO, SANTOS, 2010).

Incontinence is a problem that generates not only physiological consequences, but also psychological and social ones, as it is a problem that generates embarrassment and shame, which is why it is necessary for the professional to establish a bond, respecting and providing an opportunity for interaction with the patient (HONORIO, SANTOS, 2010).

According to the *International Continence* Society, urinary incontinence (UI) is defined as a condition in which there is involuntary loss of urine, which generates a social or hygienic problem (VALENQA et al 2016, p.44). The nurse's intervention makes it possible to recognize the needs that urinary incontinent patients have and thus contributes to the professional being able to establish the necessary care for their treatment (MATA et al, 2014).

Among the many forms of treatment for UI, we can mention pelvic floor training, biofeedback and behavioral changes (HONORIO, SANTOS, 2010). According to Valenpa et al (2016), studies show that nursing care can be divided into 4 categories:

Health Education: includes support that helps patients to carry out self-care, so that the process of "coping, rehabilitation, adaptation and acceptance of treatment" is better adhered to (VALENQA et al, 2016, p. 47). Studies also point out that this can improve self-esteem, independence and social interaction (LOCKS, 2013);

Psycho-emotional support: "IU has a negative influence on the emotional, sexual, social and psychological life of the partners of incontinent individuals" (VALENQA et al, 2016, p. 47). It is clear that there is a need not only to take care of the physical aspect, but it is also important to think about the psychosocial aspect, as it is very common to report "embarrassment, fear, changes in behavior and lifestyle in the face of UI (MATA et al, 2014, p. 3194). It is also worth remembering that taking part in support groups to share experiences is interesting for this audience and needs to be encouraged by nurses (VALENQA et al, 2016).

Behavioral treatment: a technique that makes it possible to change the patient's habits in order to improve urine loss. Among the changes are dietary habits (HONORIO, SANTOS, 2010). Changes in behavior and lifestyle, encouraging physical exercise, reducing body weight and strengthening pelvic floor muscles (VALENQA et al, 2016).

Systematization of nursing care: this highlights nursing consultations as a means of investigation, care planning, support in making decisions about treatment, monitoring the family, a time to assess changes in lifestyle, drawing up individual and specific care plans (VALENQA et al, 2016).

Given the possible alternatives for the treatment of UI in a non-surgical, non-pharmacological and non-invasive way, these alternatives can be carried out by ET:

Micturition diary and programmed urination: the former is of the utmost importance to nurses as a means of better assessing and intervening during and after treatment. It "provides important information such as urinary and water intake habits, volume ingested as well as eliminated, thus also helping to identify the type of incontinence" (LOCKY, 2013, p.43). Scheduled urination, on the other hand, is a way of guiding and modifying the urination pattern, encouraging patients to schedule their visits to the toilet (LOCKY, 2013).

Modifications to the environment and clothing: in order to list the structural aspects of the bathroom space, it needs to be as accessible as possible in order to reduce obstacles that could hinder movement, such as objects in the way. The room should be bright, clean and have an air outlet. What's more, to improve patient safety, the use of grab rails and non-slip floors provides better support and access to the bathroom. With regard to the clothing of patients with urinary urgency, it is preferable to use clothing that is easy to open and remove (LOCKY, 2013).

Food and water intake: patients should be encouraged to change their eating habits, as some foods are known to irritate the bladder and this can compromise leakage, such as caffeinated drinks, carbonated soft drinks, acidic foods, sausages and spicy foods. It is also important to reinforce water intake, as this will also contribute to proper bowel function, avoiding problems such as constipation, in combination with fiber intake and having fixed times for bowel movements (LOCKS, 2013).

Perineal exercises: these are exercises that will help consolidate the pelvic muscles, thereby increasing periurethral resistance, making it possible to reduce or eliminate urinary leakage. They are exercises that consist of "contraction and relaxation of the pelvic floor muscles, for pre-oriented times and intervals" (LOCKS, 2013, p. 45).

Biofeedback: "This is a demonstrative teaching method based on a computerized instrument that can be used to help the patient perform and contract the perineal muscles correctly" (LOCKS, 2013, p. 45).

Perineal exercises with resistance: these are exercises performed with a support of vaginal cones "which are the same size but with different weights. They help develop awareness of how to correctly contract and support the perineal muscles" (LOCKS, 2013, p. 45).

Vaginal/anal electrostimulation - the contraction of the perineal muscles is carried out through "electrical stimulation, passively and involuntarily, through the placement of a vaginal or even anal transducer. These stimuli help to strengthen the pelvic muscles and inhibit involuntary detrusor contractions" (LOCKS, 2013, p. 45-6).

The treatment options for UI are varied, and the ET should acquire all the necessary knowledge about the techniques and equipment that exist. It's important to encourage self-care, because if the patient is active throughout the treatment process and makes the necessary changes, it's easier for them to adapt and the professional should just be the facilitator of the procedure (HONORIO; SANTOS, 2010).

According to Souza (2015, p. 23), "anal incontinence (AI) is defined as the involuntary loss of feces or gas, at any time in life after learning to use the toilet", the person loses the ability to physiologically control in a socially appropriate place and time.

The causes that can generate an AI in an individual are variable, but it is important to remember that this "functional alteration can generate insecurity, loss of self-esteem, anguish, depression, physical, mental and social disorders, which contribute to a worsening in the individual's quality of life" (SOUZA, 2015, p.25). All these reactions happen because, like UI, it is a situation that generates embarrassment and shame.

It's important to remember that the pH of feces is "capable of damaging the skin", which is why ET requires constant concern for the skin, so that it doesn't end up developing skin lesions from being in constant contact with feces (SOUZA, 2015). "It is necessary to examine the condition of the skin and the surgical wound and the existence of complications" (YAMADA et al, 2009, digital text). Dermatitis is common, "conceived as areas of erythema and oedema located on the surface of the skin, which may or may not be accompanied by bullous lesions, exudate, erosion or secondary skin infection" (SOUZA, 2015, p.26).

As a treatment, patients "first have the option of conservative treatment (sacral nerve stimulation or biofeedback therapy) and then surgical treatment (sphincteroplasty)" (SOUZA, 2015, p.94). The type of treatment will depend on "the integrity of the anal sphincter".

It is interesting to note that nursing care for this public has a lot to do with the ability to positively stimulate patients, as they deal with many situations of sadness, anger or frustration. It is necessary to contribute to "re-establishing the balance between the individual with himself, with the other and with the environment in which he finds himself" (SOUZA, 2015, p.95). The value of participating in self-help groups should be "emphasized" (YAMADA et al, 2009, digital text).

ET care covers the pre-operative period, the intra-operative period, the immediate and immediate post-operative period and the late post-operative period. It is always necessary to carry out the nursing consultation implementing the SNC, as this will make it possible to systematize care. Home visits, when necessary, are also important (YAMADA et al, 2009).

It is interesting to note that in the preoperative period, the patient needs to be "instructed on the surgical procedure, prior preparation in general, the use of catheters and various collection equipment and public assistance programs" (YAMADA et al, 2009, digital text). Always prioritizing self-care and promoting rehabilitation.

5 FINAL CONSIDERATIONS

From the study carried out, it is clear that stomatherapy is a branch of nursing specialization with major challenges. The historical findings prove that its origins are quite old and that over time this specialization has gained space and prominence.

The number of people undergoing intestinal detour is growing every day, which is why we can see how important ET is, as it actively participates in the whole process of rehabilitating these people. We also know that the number of people with wounds or incontinence is also high, once again confirming its importance.

It is worth emphasizing that stomatherapy nursing care contributes significantly to the improvement of these patients, as it is a professional trained to deal with these types of problems. The study clearly showed the various roles of ET and how they should act in each situation.

We have proven all of our objectives set out in the research project, such as: identifying the role of the ET nurse, looking for all the advances in care, showing that they are primarily responsible for various procedures such as health promotion, prevention and rehabilitation, which is one of the fundamental roles of the ET nurse.

It's worth remembering that the OT must assume their role within the multidisciplinary team, contributing to the patient's care plan and that they must exercise their autonomy and carry out all their duties with responsibility and competence.

The study also showed that the ET is the main advisor and must teach and stimulate self-care for these patients, their functions are not limited to just performing a dressing, but encompass the patient in all their physical, emotional and social aspects.

Finally, we hope that this work will be a reflection for all health professionals, especially nurses, so that it can be an incentive for future new research on the subject, since it is so important and due to the scarcity of current publications.

6 REFERENCES

BRAZIL, **Ministry of Health**. Ordinance No. 620, of November 12, 2010. Table of Brazilian Classification of Occupations used in SCNES, CBOs 2231 - G1 - INTERVENTION CARDIOLOGIST MEDICIAN, 3222 - E3 - PERFUSIONIST TECHNICIAN and STOMATHERAPIST NURSE. Available at: <http://bvsms.saude.Qov.br/bvs/saudeleQis/sas/2010/prt0620 12 112010 .html> Accessed on September 29, 2016.

BRITO, K. K. G. de. Chronic wounds: nursing approach in postgraduate scientific production. **Rev enferm UFPE on line**, Recife, 2013, p. 414-21. Available at: <http://www.revista.ufpe.br/revistaenfermagem/index.php/revista/article/download/34 32/5310> Accessed on: 15 Apr. 2017.

BORGES, E. L. The role of nurses in stomatherapy and Brazilian legislation: advances and growth in the field. **Rev. Enferm. Cent. O. Min. (RECON)**, v.6. n.2. mai/ago 2016. Available at: <http://www.seer.ufsj.edu.br/index.php/recom/article/view/1467/1112> Accessed on: September 19, 2016.

CAMPOS, A. A. G. de (coord.); MORE, L. F. (org.); ARRUDA, S. S. de (org.). **Wound care protocol**. Florianopolis. Municipal Health Department, 2006. Available at: <http://www.pmf.sc.qov.br/arquivos/arquivos/pdf/26 10 2009 10.46.46.f3edcb3b301c 541c121c7786c676685d.pdf> Accessed on 22 Apr. 2017.

CARNEIRO, C. M.; SOUSA, F. B. de; GAMA, F. N. Wound treatment: nursing care in primary health care units. **Revista Enfermagem Integrada**, Ipatinga: Unileste-MG, v.3, n.2, 2010, p. 494-505. Available at:https://www.unilestemg.br/enfermagemintegrada/artigo/V3 2/03-tratamento-de-ferias-assitencia-de-enfermagem.pdf> Accessed on: 15 abr. 2107.

CARVALHO, V. M. J.; CARDOSO, J. R. da S. Care of peristomal dermatitis. In: MALAGUTTI, William; KAKIHARA, Cristiano Tarzio (org.). **Dressings, ostomy and dermatology**: a multiprofessional approach. Sao Paulo: Martinari, 2014.

CESARETTI, I.U. R.; LEITE, M. das G. Bases for care in stomatherapy. In: SANTOS, Vera Lucia Conceigao de Gouveia; CESARETTI, Isabel Umbelina Ribeiro. **Assistance in stomatherapy: caring for people with stomas**. Sao Paulo: Atheneu, 2015.

COSTA, C. R. de L.; BRITO, B. V. de; COSTA, M. M. L. Rediscovering dressing: correlation between technical/scientific preparation and the relevance of nursing autonomy in stomatherapy. In: 17° SENPE SEMINARIO NACIONAL DE PESQUISA EM ENFERMAGEM, 2013, Natal. **Electronic proceedings**... Natal, 2013. Available at: <

http://www.abeneventos.com.br/anaissenpe/17senpe/pdf/1274po.pdf> Accessed on:

23 Sept. 2016.

DIAS, M. de S. C.; PAULA, M. A. B. de; MORITA, A. B. P. da S. Perfil Profissional de Enfermeiros Estomaterapeutas Egressos da Universidade de Taubate. **Rev. ESTIMA**, v.12, n.3, 2014. Available at: <http://www.revistaestima.com.br/index.php/estima/article/view/92> Accessed on: September 20, 2016.

FRANQA, N. A. da S. et al. Acute and chronic wounds: a bibliographic review in search of evidence for care. In: VI CONCCEPAR: Scientific Congress of the Central-Western Region of Paraná. 2015. Campo Mourao. **Electronic proceedings**... Campo Mourao, 2015. Available at: http://conccepar2015.grupointegrado.br/resumo/feridas-agudas-e-cronicas-uma-revisao-bibliografica-na-busca-de-evidencias-para-o-cuidado/640> Accessed on: 18 Apr. 2017.

FERREIRA, A. M.; CANDIDO, M. C. F. da S.; CANDIDO, M. A. O cuidado de pacientes com feridas e a construgao da autonomia do enfermeiro. Rio de Janeiro: **Rev. enferm. UERJ**, 2010, p. 656-60. Available at <http://www.facenf.uerj.br/v18n4/v18n4a26.pdf> Accessed on: September 20, 2016.

HONORIO, M. O.; SANTOS, S. M. A. dos. The support network for incontinent patients: the search for support and treatment. **Rev. enferm. UERJ**, Rio de Janeiro, 2010, p. 383-8. Available at: <http://www.facenf.uerj.br/v18n3/v18n3a08.pdf> Accessed on April 19, 2017.

LOCKS, M. O. H. **Urinary incontinence in hospitalized elderly women**: challenges for nursing care. 2013. 179 f. Thesis (Doctorate in Nursing) - Health Sciences Center - Federal University of Santa Catarina, Florianopolis. 2013. Available at: <https://repositorio.ufsc.br/> Accessed on: Apr. 10, 2017.

MATA, L. R. F. da. National scientific production in nursing journals related to urinary incontinence: an integrative review. **Rev enferm UFPE online**. Recife, 2014, p. 3188-96. Available at: <http://www.revista.ufpe.br/revistaenfermagem/index.php/revista/article/download/553 3/10309> Accessed on: April 20, 2017.

MITTAG, B. F. et al. Skin lesion care: nursing augurs. **Rev. ESTIMA**, v.15, n.1,2017, p. 19-25. Available at: <https://www.revistaestima.com.br/index.php/estima/article/view/447> Accessed on: 15 Apr. 2017.

MORAIS, D. An **ostomized woman can you keep the charm**: ostomy. Goiania, 4 ed, 2009, p. 9-10. Available at: <http://www.abraso.org.br/cart ostomized woman 4ed.pdf> Accessed on: 14 Apr. 2017.

OROSCO, S. S.; MARTINS, E. A. P. Evaluating wounds: a description for systematizing care. **Rev. Enfermagem Brasil**, n.1, 2006. Available at: <http://www.faculdadesmonteneQro.edu.br/Enfermaqem 2006.pdf#page=45> Accessed on: Apr. 22, 2017.

PAULA, M. A. B. de; SANTOS, V. L. C. de G. O significado de ser especialista para o enfermeiro estomaterapeuta. **Rev. Latino - am Enfermagem**, 2003, p. 474-82. Available at: <http://www.scielo.br/scielo.php?script=sci arttext&pid=S010411692003000400010> Accessed on: September 22, 2016.

ROCHA, J. J. R. da. Intestinal stomas (ileostomies and colostomies) and intestinal anastomoses. In: SIMPOSIO FUNDAMENTOS EM CLINICA CIRURGICA, 3. ed, v.44, n. 1, cap. v, 2011, p. 51 -6. Ribeirao Preto. **Proceedings**... Sao Paulo: USP, 2011. Available at: <http://revista.fmrp.usp.br/2011/vol44n1/Simp5 Stomas%20intestinal.pdf> Accessed on: 14 Apr. 2017.

RODRIGUES, A. B. et al. **O guia da enfermagem**: fundamentos para assistência. Sao Paulo: Iatria, 2008.

SANTOS, V. L. C. de Gouveia. Stomatherapy through the ages. In: SANTOS, Vera Lucia Conceigao de Gouveia; CESARETTI, Isabel Umbelina Ribeiro. **Assistance in stomatherapy: caring for people with stomas**. Sao Paulo: Atheneu, 2015.

SILVA, F. A. A. et al. Nursing in stomatherapy: clinical care for patients with venous ulcers. **Rev. Bras. Enferm,** Brasilia, 2009, p. 889-93. Available at: <http://www.scielo.br/pdf/reben/v62n6/a14v62n6> Accessed on: 22 Apr. 2017.

SOUZA, L. C. de. **Anal incontinence and nursing diagnosis**: determinants, prevalence and social representations. 2015. 129 f. Dissertation (Master's in Nursing) - Technology, Culture and Communication in Health and Nursing - TECCSE - Federal University of Juiz de Fora, Juiz de Fora, 2015. Available at: <https://repositorio.ufjf.br/jspui/bitstream/ufjf/341/1/lucienecarnevaledesouza.pdf> Accessed on: 10 Apr. 2017

SOUZA, N. Z. de et al. The role of nurses in the stomatherapy service. In: II JORNADA INTERNACIONAL DE ENFERMAGEM VISIBILIDADE PROFESSIONAL DO ENFERMEIRO: avangos e conquistas, 2. ed. 2012, Santa Maria. **Electronic proceedings**... Santa Maria, 2012. Available at: <http://www.unifra.br/eventos/jornadadeenfermagem/Trabalhos/4256.pdf> Accessed on: April 20, 2017.

TEIXEIRA, A. K. S.; MENEZES, L. C. G. de; OLIVEIRA, R. M. Stomatherapy service from the perspective of nursing managers in a public referral hospital. **Rev. ESTIMA**, v.14, n.1,2016, p. 3-12. Available at: <http://webcache.googleusercontent.com/search?q=cache:v6RdHBADGK0J:www.rev istaestima.com.br/index.php/estima/article/download/114/pdf+&cd=1&hl=en-BR&ct=clnk&gl=br> Accessed on: September 19, 2016.

VALENQA, M. P. et al. Nursing care in urinary incontinence: an integrative review study. **Rev. ESTIMA**, v.14, n.1, 2016, p. 43-9. Available at: <https://www.revistaestima.com.br/index.php/estima/article/view/195/pdf> Accessed on: 15 Apr. 2017.

VASCONCELLOS, F. M.; XAVIER, Z. D. M. The nurse in the care of the colostomized client based on Orem's theory. **Revista Recien**. Sao Paulo, 2015, p. 2537. Available at: <http://www.recien.com.br/index.php/Recien/article/view/108/176> Accessed on: April 19, 2017.

YAMADA, B. F. A. Stomatherapy - history. **Brazilian Association of Stomatherapy: stomata, wounds and incontinence**. Available at: <http://www.sobest.org.br/texto/6> Accessed on: September 21, 2016.

YAMADA, B. F. A., ROGENSKI, N. M. B.; OLIVEIRA, P. de A. Aspectos historicos, eticos e legais da estomaterapia. **Rev. ESTIMA**, v.1, n.2, 2003. Available at: <http://www.revistaestima.com.br/index.php/estima/article/view/130> Accessed on: September 21, 2016.

YAMADA, B. F. A. et al. **Stomatherapy - competencies of the stomatherapist nurse Ti SOBEST or the stomatherapist nurse**. 2009. Available at: <http://www.sobest.org.br/texto/11> Accessed on September 27, 2016.

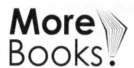
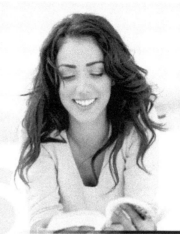

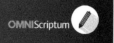

Milton Keynes UK
Ingram Content Group UK Ltd.
UKHW011147010424
440421UK00001B/339